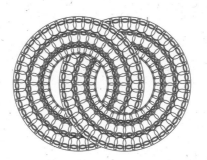

But I Still Have
My Fingerprints

But I
Still Have My
Fingerprints

Dianne
Silvestri, MD

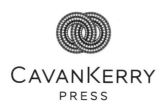

CAVANKERRY
PRESS

CavanKerry Press Ltd.
Fort Lee, New Jersey
www.cavankerrypress.org

Publisher's Cataloging-In-Publication Data
(Prepared by The Donohue Group, Inc.)
Names: Silvestri, Dianne, author.
Title: But I still have my fingerprints / Dianne Silvestri, MD.
Description: First edition. | Fort Lee, New Jersey : CavanKerry Press, 2022.
Identifiers: ISBN 9781933880945
Subjects: LCSH: Silvestri, Dianne—Poetry. | Acute myeloid leukemia—Patients—
    Poetry. | Women physicians—Poetry. | Stem cells—Transplantation—Poetry. | Acute
    myeloid leukemia—Chemotherapy—Poetry. | LCGFT: Autobiographical poetry.
Classification: LCC RC643 .S55 2022 | DDC 616.994190092—dc23

Cover artwork: Ron Mellott / Stocksy United
Cover and interior text design by Ryan Scheife, Mayfly Design
First Edition 2022, Printed in the United States of America

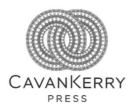

 Made possible by funds from the New Jersey State Council on the Arts, a partner agency of the National Endowment for the Arts.

CavanKerry Press is grateful for the support it receives from the New Jersey State Council on the Arts.

In addition, CavanKerry Press gratefully acknowledges generous emergency support received during the COVID-19 pandemic from the following funders:

The Academy of American Poets

Community of Literary Magazines and Presses

The Mellon Foundation

National Book Foundation

New Jersey Arts and Culture Recovery Fund

New Jersey Council for the Humanities

New Jersey Economic Development Authority

Northern New Jersey Community Foundation

The Poetry Foundation

US Small Business Administration

Also by Dianne Silvestri, MD

Necessary Sentiments (2015)

Dedicated to the loving One

who made the me that was

and the me that is.

Endurance won't
be enough, though without it
you can't get to the place
where more of you is asked.

—Stephen Dunn

Contents

Time Out

Runoff

Foreword

I have had the great privilege of caring for this remarkable physician, patient, and poet whose words describing her journey confronting acute leukemia grace these pages. I am a hematologist oncologist specializing in blood cancers and bone marrow transplantation, working hand in hand with a wonderfully dedicated and devoted team. We meet people at a time of personal existential threat, creating an intimate connection with patients and their families in their time of need. We are given a unique window into their moments of courage, fear, disappointment, and perseverance. As caregivers, we are confronted by uncertainty and vulnerabilities that we all share. This reality is often brought home with a greater sense of immediacy when caring for medical personnel who have been struck by illness.

Acute myeloid leukemia is a life-threatening cancer of the blood. It often appears without warning and can present with symptoms of tiredness, fever, bruising, or bleeding. The diagnosis is rendered without much warning: examination of the blood under the microscope in the emergency room calls attention to this possibility, and a subsequent bone marrow examination provides confirmation. The patient is shortly confronted with the imminency of the danger. Protective steps are required to prevent life-threatening consequences. Chemotherapy is initiated in patients who are able to tolerate the side effects, with the goal of killing the leukemia cells in the bone marrow and allowing for healthy blood cells to return. This period involves close monitoring in the hospital through many weeks and is characterized by low blood counts, creating a significant risk for infection and the need for transfusions of red blood cells and platelets. If patients demonstrate recovery of normal blood counts, without evidence of persistent leukemia, they are considered to be in complete remission. Additional therapy is then needed to eliminate disease that is not visible, with the hope of subsequently achieving a cure. This second step may involve a bone marrow transplant from a matched donor in which the immune system that is transferred potentially displaces any remaining leukemia cells with donor-derived blood production. This process involves considerable risk from infection as the donor immune system learns to protect the recipient, while avoiding excess immune response that can target normal tissues, a phenomenon called graft vs. host disease.

Dianne's poetry powerfully illuminates the depth and complexity of her feelings during this journey. Her first poems belie a surreal sense of disconnection and alienation from the diagnosis and its consequences. In "The Night Phlebotomist," she poignantly describes her sense of complete vulnerability and loss of control. In "Doctor as Patient," she shares the feelings and altered perspective that accompany this dramatic change in roles. A dermatologist by training, she writes personally about her experience of hair loss and speaks intimately of picking out a head covering with her husband. "Conversation with My Grandson" brings together the innocent directness of questions of life and death with her navigation between hope and uncertainty. She marvels at the connection with the young male donor whose immunity now courses through her veins hopefully bringing protection and not danger. As she perseveres through her journey and questions the nature of hope, she prevails, reconciling loss with the joy of survival, appreciating the unique privilege of hope and anticipation for the future.

Through the immediacy of feeling that characterizes her work, Dianne's remarkable strength and honesty shine through. Her illness strips away her sense of safety and the protective layer of her professional life, forcing her to confront the ephemeral nature and uncertainty of life. She does not avert her eyes but courageously probes deeply into her feelings and discovers beauty, wisdom, and meaning as she navigates and finds hope. Through the many years I have been her caregiver, she has taught me a sense of wonder toward the possibilities of the human spirit.

David Avigan, MD
Chief, Division of Hematology and Hematologic Malignancies
Beth Israel Deaconess Medical Center
Codirector, Immunotherapy Institute
Rosenberg Clinical Cancer Center
Professor of Medicine
Harvard Medical School

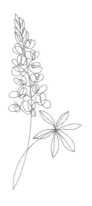

Dear Doctor

Emergency Phone Call from My Doctor, 11pm

You have almost no white cells.
Through encore ER appraisals,
enclosed and exposed by scraping
metal curtain rings,
I endure for the verdict at dawn:
more defenseless than dangerous.

They belt me to a gurney to jolt
into an ambulance vault
where six spotlights drill through me
from the quilted stainless-steel ceiling.
During transfer the uniformed man
taps a clipboard, makes small talk,

but the surreal all-nighter has drugged me.
He swirls my cart through corridors,
triggers open automatic doors,
and rolls me under the banner
announcing my unthinkable deposit
on the seventh-floor tower of leukemics.

Cosmic Questions

I learned of a man in a Bosnian town
    who, rather than rant and curse,

purchased steel plates for his roof
    after scientists verified

the sixth meteor strike in three years.
    Experts cannot explain

this homing of galactic trash
    to a tiny terrestrial target,

nor do they understand
    why one of my white cells turned killer.

Daunorubicin

You save lives, you take them.
Your methods I memorized
from the thick blue textbook,
a cruelty still vivid.

You're Dr. Jekyll and Mr. Hyde,
but I have no choice.
My tears cannot bargain.
I clutch my son's hand,

beg God for mercy
as the nurse clocks her push
on the big-barreled plunger
to send your scourge tunneling

to my core to assassinate
all proliferating cells.
Oh, crimson savage,
leave me alive!

Chemotherapy

Here, on the far
side of the moon, it's all
dead reckoning, the end
of night blown
from sight. Shifting
infinitude scours away
my barefoot prints.

I must
be transfiguring
into heavy ashes
for a maroon velvet
bag, my only
need, a gold
braided drawstring.

The floor is too cold,
too hard to kneel,
but hear me,
God. Hold me.

The Night Phlebotomist

The corridors seethe with nocturnal predators,
their voices low.

My door latch coughs, a figure hisses,
I've come to draw blood,

wrenches my arm like a lamb shank,
rasps it with alcohol, plunges her spike,

pops one color-coded, rubber-stoppered
vial after another into the sheath,

unplugs each loaded one to add
to the crimson log pile weighting my thigh,

steals more, it seems, than ought to be ample
from this provisional liquor of my life.

Doctor as Patient

In medical school
we all imagined

catching infirmities
as we learned them—

Addison's, myxedema.
Every headache:

a brain tumor.
I'm now awkwardly

beached, my white coat
surrendered, modesty

breached by the gaping
leak of the extra-

large blue gown
as students file in.

I agree to be
their mannequin,

let them interview me,
smile and survey,

palpate, percuss,
and auscultate me,

because I recall
my young stethoscope

on early test runs.
Now ripped from my role

as teaching *physician*,
I body-double

as teaching *case*,
naked in a snow globe.

For the Patients with Hair Loss

I reassure the ones who lose:
once handfuls shed, hair will regrow.
A few months' patience pays the dues.

Scalp hair growth reacts to clues
but resumes its cycle status quo,
I reassure the ones who lose.

But now *my* fiberglass unglues,
clots choke my hairbrush post-chemo.
A few months' patience should pay the dues.

I give my son scissors to use,
but after the trim, more bare spots show.
I'm now among the ones who lose.

Webs colonize the room. I choose
to be buzzed bald, accept the glow
and hope my patience will pay the dues.

This familiar voice dealt rosy news,
but its face in the mirror I do not know.
I once reassured others who lose,
but will patience really pay *my* dues?

Skullcap

Ron pushes the wheelchair
to the gift shop for me
to find a skullcap,
something soft
to cushion the bare shock
and warm my head at night.

He tells me I look beautiful,
even half-hidden
by the pleated mask,
and says I won't need
a wig, the hair will
grow back soon enough,

but adds, I should try on
the coral-checked sunhat
that will be cute for summer.

Poem for George

I've named this special IV pole George,
my constant companion in empty hours
through chemo and the eternal waiting.

He tirelessly suspends fluid balloons
and supports pumps that purr and sizzle
like dizzy bees pushing mysteries into me.

George is strong to steady my step
and sometimes winks his gleam at my gloom.
He doesn't object if I push him away

when I need some space. Infrequently
his tires accidentally roll over the three
trailing tubes that hitch us together.

He tries to fit his six-wheeled stance
beside the toilet in my narrow bathroom.
He's become a friend, even if twice

he nipped my ankle, but I understand—
my anger slips out sometimes too.

A Bag of Blood

In med school I reclined once every
    three months on blood bank vinyl

as a rocking plastic canister
    tick-tocked, tapping a warm river

that coursed from my open arm—
    a stress-free deed I exchanged

for a stipend of twenty-five dollars
    to ease my austere living,

not once making the visit graphic
    as if possibly paying it forward.

The Hospital Mail

At no particular hour
the door to my room snaps open
to a snuffling yellow paper gown
wearing an orange pleated mask

and extending a rubber-gloved fistful
of mail—envelopes penned
with my name, sealed 2-D visitors
stolen in to console me.

Care bleeds from the ink,
otherwise impotent
to effect *Get well soon!*
or abracadabra *Feel strong!*

I split the silence open.
Neither of us has words
to ensure I will improve
or admit I may not survive.

Hospital Housekeeping

May I clean your room?
Oh yes . . . and not just this one.
Please go on to all those
at home I cannot get to,
the overstuffed drawers,
my yellowed stamp collection,
oversized box of Palm Island
seashells beached on the top shelf,
and stashes of guilt from college.

All done with this meal tray?
Oh yes . . . and completely
exhausted of all desire.

Aubade

Daybreak crawls in scarred,
the sky thick enough to shovel.
Below my window the roof

of the parking garage is empty
for repairs. A jackhammered crater
plugged with a rust-spattered plate

is being patched with cement
smoothed like putty in a nail hole.
The garage across Binney Street

winds full of pickup trucks
first to the sky-view deck,
joined by a crawl of cars

jostling Rubik's-like,
pull aside, let pass, advance,
a game I observe without playing.

Conversation with My Grandson

Grandie,

        what do you think happens

    the moment you die?

           Does *real* you fly away?

Will you still be able to see me down here?

      Do you think you'll hear if I talk to you?

Will it be cold   like outer space

               or hot . . .

      so high and close to the sun?

Will there be a swimming pool?

      Can angels swim?

        Or do wings melt in water?

What do you think God will say

        when you get there?

Seated on My Hospital Bed

My seventh-floor window vibrates.
      The room throbs in crescendo
as a rescue helicopter stitches
      a curved seam across the sky
bound for Children's Hospital.
      Balanced like a dragonfly,
it settles on the roof.
      As the blades stretch to slow,
curled jumpsuits spring free,
      deliver a cot, coax it up
to stand on baby deer legs,
      urge it toward a door.
My mind draws in close,
      imagining the injured child
or fevered unconscious body,
      the nearby ashen parents.
I blink. My self-pity has vanished.

Bone Marrow Biopsy

Days drag past since the needle pressed
into my core, its suction gurgling.

Experts weigh if my disease is banished,
dissect the slush and extracted spicules

like when we tweezed owl pellets in fifth grade
to untangle the remnants of a mouse, a bat,

a small bird with claws preserved,
submitted the disarticulated tally

logged from the owl's expectorated dross,
sobering evidence of life sacrificed

in natural selection. I wonder if the news
will relegate me to join the world's refuse.

The wait is so long. I touch my hip
still tender from the doctor's drill.

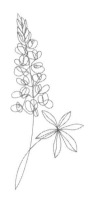

Off Script

Donor Search

My sister and I used to play
we were teachers recording grades
or secretaries filing or mothers tending
babies and frying rubber eggs
or clerks ringing grocery sales to each other
on our red plastic cash register.

I held her hand to cross the driveway
to Sylvia's house or the neighbor boys'.
She taught me all she learned in school.
We sat wedged on the bench for piano duets.

I hesitate to phone her now,
don't want to tell her the results disclose
she cannot be my marrow donor.
Like piano keys, the black and white
stripes on her sixth chromosome
are an exact match to mine except

for a single rare shift in the embryo
of one of us.

Dear Healthy 28-Year-Old Man

How did you get the idea
to be a marrow donor?

What prompted you to sign
to let them swab your cheek?

Why did you take a chance
somewhere there might be a me?

How did you feel when they called
to warn you could be a match?

Did they ask if you still meant it,
still wanted to give your cells?

How did you react when your blood
confirmed your chromosome for immunity

was a picture of the totem of mine?
Ten stripes in perfect match.

Did you know about the shots
that would drive your bones to ache

to make newborn cells to be siphoned,
sifted, and shipped on ice

to me, longing, readied, and waiting?
Whoever you are,

will your sacrifice be worthwhile?

Isolation Room, Leukemia Floor

Entry proceeds through successive air-locked
   chambers with heavy sucking doors.

Weapons are exiled—not guns and knives,
    but microbes. Only unopened toothpaste,

soap, and shampoo, sanitary scalded
   clothing sealed in plastic bags.

The admitting nurse swabs disinfectant
   over everything else headed inbound.

I strip off street clothes; light blue is the new orange.
   Attendants don masks and gowns, rubber gloves,

as if what's left of me is contagious.
   I beg to be spared the hard, cold floor

in standard-issue gripper socks.
   They frown but agree to inspect my shoebox,

nod their approval of my freshly-purchased,
   white-laced sneakers with aster pink soles,

hot aqua fenders—consoling vestige
   to show I am me.

Countdown to a New Birthday

The transplant team rehearses, nurses
cheery, my doctor wearing grave hope.

From Day Minus Seven, they all engage
the protocol for Conditioning Week.
I sign consent for alien infusions
with extra-long names and side effects.

They admit no one knows what will happen.
I take the swishes, pills, swallows,
designed to disarm all resistance
not already drained by my terror.

Day Minus Five I lose count
to severe infection, poisoned gut,
drowning lungs, caretaker panic.
I hear a buzzing all-night movie
of bright-colored swirling chips,
snaking chutes, a cable unraveling
a giant steel ball.
                     Once, on Day Zero,
I open my eyes to a plastic tube of pink
sludge of stem cells coming to strike me
with shakes and aches, a nurse shouting, *Morphine.*

Three days later I wake to unknown
people who gush how improved I look.
My husband's face unfolds a smile.

Awaiting Reconstitution

I am now my proxy,
a mirage of me
swirling with sap
of a different DNA,
my vacant marrow
waiting for adopted
cells to populate,
maybe tomorrow,
while I pray for a truce
between genomes
who quarrel like siblings.

Rescued, yes,
but confined, too strained
to name it repose,
more like perpetually
renewed postponement,
endless intermission,
my life
locked out.

Swallow This

Rx: Take one Magic School Bus ride
    to watch your chalky, boxy tablet
    swallowed three times a day pivot
    crosswise in flow to crash the wall.

Rx: Feel the girth of your dime-sized disc
    guaranteed to provoke a choke.

Rx: Taste these five tiny pills at once
    to learn they're bitter as a kumquat.

Rx: Try that shiny, twice-a-day capsule
    to note its size like a mobile home
    requires a great gulp of ginger ale
    and nearly always a second effort,
    then trails the potent stench of skunk.

Chimera

*chimera, n.: an organism with tissues of diverse genetic
composition; a fanciful or nearly impossible idea*

There's a man in my life,
nesting in caverns in my bones,

pulsing his excursions,
and navigating forks in my veins,

almost as if he owns them.
The blood in there I call *mine*,

but its cells wear *his* signature.
I pray this union will work,

but worry about a mutiny.
I must find a way to persuade

the new guy to be my ally.
God, help the two of me get along.

Drug-Induced Tendon Tear

In eighth-grade art class
we sat at long tables
slathering sloppy strips
of torn paper

over an old light bulb
to mold a puppet head.
Mine stared from beneath
heavy brows,

smiled fat sausage lips
like a crazed uncle.
A horseshoe of glued yarn
skirted his bald pate.

Today, in the cast room,
I ponder my puppet's
earlier personae,
ones buried as I mashed

each layer over the last
to change the chin,
regroove the forehead,
resculpt the nose

and cheeks, reshape
his lips to be broader,
choose the width
of his gaze. The head

scarred hard in drying,
earlier visages covered,
just like former me,
smothered, gone.

Demolition

From inside the windows
of my isolation room

I monitor Jurassic progress
in the drama across the street.

Early each weekday morning
hard hats invade like beetles.

One climbs the excavator,
annoys its neck to straighten

and reach for the aging gymnasium,
spread wide its pincer to bite

another free edge to splinter
the black roof, leaving gnarled

girders like tough spaghetti
stuck in the raptor's teeth.

Cement and brick walls crumble
under the champing jaw.

I barely move from the scene
when my nurse brings a meal of pills.

Suddenly the mean head tilts,
smirks a sideways glance

directly at my face
as if spying his dessert.

Advance Directive

If I don't come home from the light
   blue walls of this place, it's not

that I want to abandon you
   to do everything alone,

but don't forget to replace
   my voice with yours at home

on the answering machine.
   Please take the gourmet cooking class

you always said you wanted,
   and if you resume dance lessons,

pretend it is I waltzing with you.

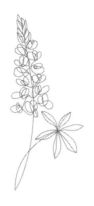

Time Out

After a Month Away

Back at my address
      azaleas devour each other,

weeds rip the sidewalk,
      laurel swarms the doorstep,

spindle trees lap the top floor,
      barberry thorns rake the sky.

I'm crazed to grab my familiar
      shears, gloves, trowel,

but soil harbors lethal spores—
      all of it off-limits.

It Would Be So Nice to Have

a Geiger counter-like gadget
   that would spit static as it hovers
   over food harboring microbes:
   lettuce, apples, grapes full of menace.

My detector would pop and sizzle to signify
   mold spores nestling on banana peels.

I'd hear it sputter when organisms swarm
   in a common pot that's not bubbling hot,
   like chicken soup or Cream of Wheat.

I'm sure it would crackle erratically over
   open bread, chips soiled by a cough,

and detonate at first notice of unroasted
   nuts, poultry, eggs undercooked,
   teeming with hazard and salmonellae—

a device to detect the silent food
   safe to consume: my uneasy rations.

Back Home, Day 459

The tree man has come today.
He's roped and dangling, half circus,

half dance in a leather belt,
aerial stuntman on a chain-

saw harness, nimble sculptor
to dismember her. Silence

collapses with a thud. Buzzing
halts when the boys on the ground

maneuver the swaying tangle-
free ropes to land large limbs

as delicately as marionettes.
Year after year, that box elder

stretched bold pom-poms skyward
from the middle of my summer yard,

strained gold paper currency
through the colander of fall,

and held wrought iron constancy
against cruel winter

until despair burrowed in
and changed all the locks.

Lying on the Patient History Form

The question requires I state
if I ever smoked cigarettes.
Surely my inhalations
are so remote they exceed
some statute of limitations.
I mean, any functional sequelae
of my limited exposure
would have mended long ago.

No one ever challenges,
Are you positive you didn't?
Besides, my experimentation
is excusable—my immaturity,
my curiosity, independence,
my roommate with the habit,
another friend across the hall,
the surgeon general's lack
of warning, and of course, my own
desire to be liked, and the ready
excuse if my parents questioned
my redolent jacket and hair.

I guess that means I lied
to them, too, my parents.
There were some secrets I kept.
I would have told them had I believed
their love would burn through.

Summer's Reprieve

A red flash startles—
damselflies,

gossamer-winged
dancing flutes,

but not the usual
azure hue.

They glisten, crimson
as clinic stylets,

needles hovering
without any threat,

delicately stitching
my sunlight.

Citrus aurantium

Seville orange. A small thick-rinded
citrus fruit with pocked orange skin.
Zest—bitter, tangy, sharply sour.

Adored by Brits who know to wash,
dry, slash its equator, pierce out
dozens of pectin-rich seeds to cinch
like innards in a muslin bag.

The French call the fruit *l'orange amère*,
a bit like *l'amour*, the petite glowing
lanterns conspiring to craft Grand
Marnier, triple sec, Cointreau.

The Seville orange inhabits Andalusia,
divine golden air succoring the trees.

But the fruit of romance conceals hazard:
a flavonoid within impairs the essential
enzyme metabolizing my transplant medicine,
freeing it to amass and poison my marrow.

Yet, a bit of peril, if *elected*, sounds nice!
I'll choose to savor Seville marmalade-
slathered toast tips, sip Grand Marnier
with my beloved by candlelight.
A dip in my counts won't kill me.

Graft vs. Host

I am now an implosion;
        my invited tenant, disruptive.

He inflates my skin to foam,
        burns my mouth's membranes,

sands my blinking,
        rifles my gut,

splots my hide like a leopard's.
        I never imagined such a question,

but just who is in control?
        Whose breath is on my tongue?

When I clean beneath my fingernails,
        whose cells do I quarry?

The Nurses There

always asked if I needed
anything more:
sugar packets,
bouillon sleeves,
steaming cups
of soothing green tea.

They patiently answered
my litany of questions,
inquired of the doctors,
called Food Service
on their emergency line.

They shifted the hours
of my infusions
to allow me a shower,
and pushed apart nighttime
to flush a dark channel
for me to sleep.

They laughed along
when I nicknamed my treatments
Van-Coke and *Swamp Juice*.
They offered swabs for my
ghoulmouth and swishes
for glob-clogger secretions.

Every time I'm readmitted, again,
I hug them, one by one.

Choosing the Right Pumpkin, Farm Stand, Natick, Mass.

You there,
you are the one,

you moon face
like those of us

who've been taking too much
prednisone for too long,

nubby scar
across your forehead,

dried abrasion
stubbling your chin.

You are
the wounded strong soul.

I will give you eyes
to find me likewise.

Appointment at the Oncology Clinic

This autumn my armor
                    is fenestrated
          like a rusted leaf,
                 no benefit
as I steal into the elevator
          too weakened,

when a musket-fired sneeze
                    explodes behind me
          hurling droplets
                 in turbulent clouds
suited to propel
          a menace of virions

two hundred times as far
                    as they normally float
          from standard breaths
                 now in this elevator
packed with targets
          like me.

MRI

Dejeweled, I lie,
still, eyes closed,
as the slab slides.

I remember Venice
before all this—
I'm reclining again

against my husband
in this narrow gondola,
squeezing his hand,

as we skim forward
beneath the low
arched bridge.

Feature Film: *Drug Study KEP DR78*

If I were directing this movie,
right after the litany of potential
side effects, the camera would pan
to the pills, not languid white,
but persimmon, peacock, chartreuse,
something lively, promising potency.

Participants in the study,
I'd cast automaton-like.
They'd return regularly to mark
the questionnaire, then depart
with the next aliquot of pills.

A scene at the refrigerated lab
will show the research assistants
blustering their paper gowns,
waving purple rubber gloves
to count the pills left
in bottles subjects return,
tapping keyboards to log
scores from questionnaires
surveying side effects,
indigestion, sadness, sex.

My favorite segment of the film:
one patient's flashback to childhood,
a bright glossy capsule
dropping into a basin
of water, a child wincing,
then grinning as the slicker dissolves
and a dinosaur with fearful jaw
emerges, writhing out, unfurled.

PTSD

I wear my pockets sewn closed—
unable to offer more than souvenir,
to reach, to unfold to 3-D—
strafed, blackened to silhouette.

This is not exaggeration.
I translate into meteor crater,
cicatrix cementing my crust,
tied down by the tyranny of fear.

Repair, brushfires, dousing,
rescue, surveillance, minefields,
deathblow, reprieve, ambush . . . .
No Undo option for this.

Darkroom in the Converted Laundry Room

I'd flash a beam through the negative
under the safelight's amber moon,
wave to dodge and burn in,

then whisk the sheet to the tank
to drift in the sour lagoon,
await the black-and-white dawn,

the moment to tong it out dripping
when I would study the outcome.
If it wasn't what I'd imagined,

I could always start again.

Readmitted: This Time to the Overflow Ward

*It is not necessary to accept everything as true, one must
only accept it as necessary.*
—Franz Kafka, *The Trial*

Just as I'm aching
for a warm blanket,
the new nurse coasts
into my room,
mascara so thick
I'm sure she can't see me.

She doesn't even seem
to know my name,
but holds out a loaded
cup of brown pills.

I don't need a laxative!

Oh, you should take them,
she strikes in the voice
of a dressing room attendant.
*We give them to everyone
here twice a day.
It's like a warm blanket.
Is there anything
else you need?*

You May Resume Your Normal Activities

as tolerated, they tell me on discharge,
but it's hard to reengage
(quit the cage, go onstage, own my rage).

I must hide these mulberry stains,
this shearable, translucent skin
(tissue-thin, plum cushion, battered twin),

my inner space flash-fry or cry mode,
but worst, my replaced face
(unknown phase, fallout trace, sheer disgrace),

from cortisone blown wide
to a visage I don't recognize
(rude disguise, unsought prize, close your eyes),

a two-eyed, full-bulging bowl
of yeast-risen cheek dough
(snow buffalo, scarecrow, freak show).

I howl at this moon.
What about you, abductee
(addressee, used-to-be-me)?

Please Define *Longer*

In the beginning my doctor
replied, *One year*, when I asked
how long I'd be out from work.

But, this morning my wash-up
mirror emits an alien
visage of sour hue,

drumstick clavicles, radiator
ribs. It whistles, *You look
like your Anatomy cadaver.*

As I'm here, my office dismembers
itself, fancy diplomas
step down from walls, momentous

files march toward discard,
grand books hitchhike to the library.
Framed photos scoot off my desk.

My Derm Society mug
rolls into a box. Sleeves
of monogrammed white jackets

drip over the trash bin lip.
I remember his answer continued:
One year . . . sometimes longer.

A Club for Those of Us Who Almost Died

Come, let's gather to commiserate
our losses—our jobs, our beauty,
our freedom to act spontaneously,
to travel without risks.

We'll understand each other
as we lament stunted energy
and sex that . . . well, isn't.
All the while we'll agree

that those outside our club
only marvel we still exist,
and conclude it's bliss to be alive . . .
or at least to look like it.

Readjustment to living continues
not as we imagined:
we mostly wish no change
would ever have been required.

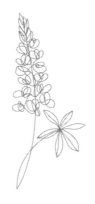

Runoff

With Feathers

The patient is at high risk of Morbidity from medications, as
well as her disease.
—my hospital chart

In Montreal with my husband,
I stroll Rue Ste-Catherine,
startle as a sidewalk sweeper
flopping his hinged dustpan
hops the curb, while the still
body of a white pigeon lies,
beak against the store's wall.

Birds that bullet my kitchen
windows may ricochet injured
but usually snap up and ruffle,
shrug off the stun and fly,
alive, maybe one feather missing.

I trouble over the on-duty doctor's
words in his note about me.
Morbidity sounds like *Mortality*.
That crimson *M* drags my neck
when I'm trying so hard to fly.

Wanted: Lust

Loss of it
is not unusual

but to lose it, unwelcome,
both of us now longing

with sighs for what
may have expired

during the long
essential diversion

as we blinked directly
into the fire,

both of us unaware
of collateral damage

as survival occupied
the sheets where we lie

in separate masks,
isolated

in sanitized insanity,
luxury stolen,

last lantern blown out,
or . . . lingering.

Flashback on a Sunny Day

The waiter brings me a baseball-
sized scoop of vanilla ice cream.

From its summit, a slow landslide
of viscous tawny caramel

sauce drifts like the same
chamois-colored slush

inched down a clear tube
into my arm from the plump

bag of blood-banked platelets,
hung to rescue me.

Rose Quartz Geode I Found in the Woods

It might crack open, that drab warty stone,
if I smacked it hard against a boulder,

might split to disclose a fist-sized cave
of sparkling crystals—flashing beauty

I only later learned was wrought
by sore time and moisture seeping

to mingle minerals in hidden space,
to squash a stack of what siphoned through cracks,

to crush and compact a scintillating marvel,
in a prolonged pinching fusion of creation,

like the ultimate reward of torment and waiting.

Maintenance Fatigue

I report back to clinic
for ever-dawning symptoms,
still-defiant ones—

this cough rocking me
like poor clutchwork.
Spasms lock my fingers

like crisscrossed crutches.
I lick clapboard lips,
blink clapboard eyes,

and wait to be wadded up
like a crossed-off calendar page.
My doctors must be ready

to abandon the stubborn enigmas
logged in my lengthening file
for a fresh, solvable case.

Although they always smile,
I know their smiles could be
just carefully taught, not true.

Waiting Room *Waiting*

I've already deleted the unwanted text
messages in my inbox, answered new ones,
sent old pics of family skin questions
into the trash. I finished reading
Kooser's *Poetry Home Repair Manual*
I brought from the library, paged through
the one available *People* magazine,
and reviewed my yawning grocery list.

I drained my water bottle an hour ago.
I am long past being tempted
to chip in on the collaborative thousand-
piece jigsaw puzzle on the table.
I know that three of its pieces are missing.
Should I try to rouse the other taxidermied
patients folded in these seats?
Could a Kozak workout save the day?

Retail Therapy

Declared fit to shop for groceries,
I heap my carriage with bulging bags,

off-load bounty to my car,
coax my empty cart on the asphalt

to surge toward the highlight of the trip.
At the return stall I plunge the cart

into the queue in clattering collision,
thrust it through the nearest basket's back,

then ram the two to engage some strays,
grating cacophony while I assemble

those flung pell-mell by odd customers
who don't appreciate how good this feels.

Victory Garden

In the glazed, teal ceramic planter
my husband received from his best friend
when I was near death,

the burgeoning Dieffenbachia
beside the red-veined prayer plant
blanches three blades weekly,

and when those leaves are lopped,
the blackening fingers of palm
deeper in the jungle wither

in ominous demise.
Plants in general are heartless.
I mean, after surviving five years,

my husband's victory garden
now threatens, and I feel I *must* keep
us both alive—for him.

An End to the Ends

I vow to resign
from mentally marking
ultimates—

last plane trip south,
last deck-flowered summer,
last days on Cape Cod,
last Christmas together.

It's time to twist
my lipstick up
for a first-ditch list,
cast my fancy
for fresh adventures—

tackle the tango,
taste more reds,
tramp a new trail
to a new museum
on a secret beach
far off in New Zealand.

New Life

Hague's Peak, Colorado

Ravenous sky-struck flames
ripped the evergreen cloak

from this mountain not long ago.
Dayglow draws me to range

its meadow, to kneel, gather
fragments of trunks, charred

spicules still tinged with smoke.
I pack them home to loop

pink and yellow ribbon
through the scorched whorls

to spangle my Christmas tree
and remind me of snow buttercups,

scarlet paintbrush, silvery
lupine emerging from the ruins.

Glossary

Addison's—The name applied to a disorder of deficiency of adrenal gland hormone production.

advance directive—A legal document that protects one's right to refuse unwanted medical interventions and to request desired treatment measures in the event one loses the capability to make those decisions.

auscultate—To listen through a stethoscope or other instrument to sounds within the body.

biopsy—To cut out a sample for examination through the microscope or other methods.

bone marrow—Tissue in the core of many bones where the production of blood cells occurs.

Conditioning Week—The time during which immunosuppressive drugs and sometimes irradiation are given to prepare a person for receiving transplantation of tissue from someone else.

Day Zero—The day of infusion or insertion of transplanted cells.

donor matching—The comparison of two individuals' immune reactivity genes, performed to find a similar donor for someone in need of cells or an organ, in an attempt to minimize both the risk that the recipient will reject the transplant and the risk the donated tissue will damage its new host. A donor is sought whose genetic code for human leukocyte antigen (HLA) resembles the recipient's as closely as possible. HLA is a protein signal present on most cells that allows the body to distinguish its own cells from those that do not belong. The genetic code for HLA markers is inherited, half from the mother and half from the father. For this reason, identical twins carry identical markers, but siblings have only a 25% chance of sharing the same genetic immune type. Transplant centers hope for a match of five different markers on each one of the pair of number 6 chromosomes: A, B, C, DRB1, and DQ. If all ten markers of the donor match the ten of the patient, it is called a perfect, or 10 of 10, match. The HLA code sites on the chromosomes are sometimes depicted by lines banding the two ribbon-like chromosomes.

genome—The unique, full set of genetic material (nucleotides) on all of a person's chromosomes.

graft—The cells, tissue, or organ of the donor infused in, implanted in, or affixed onto a person.

graft vs. host disease—A term that includes various disorders that occur after stem cells from a healthy donor are infused into the host patient. The problems are caused by the implanted immune cells attacking tissues in their new home. Signs of such injury can occur quickly (in acute or aGVHD) or develop months later (in chronic or cGVHD).

gurney—A cot on wheels, typically used to transport patients in hospitals or ambulances.

host—The recipient of transplanted cells.

immune reconstitution—Restoration of partial or complete function of the immune system after impairment from inborn defect, disease, or therapeutic destruction.

immunosuppressed—Having an immune system compromised by heredity, disease, or treatments.

MRI (magnetic resonance imaging)—A method of three-dimensional scanning that utilizes strong magnetic forces to create the image.

myxedema—A term referring to skin infiltrated with mucinous material in hypothyroidism.

percuss—To tap on a part of the body to evaluate by sound if solid, liquid, or air is beneath.

phlebotomist—An individual who removes (draws) blood samples, that is, performs phlebotomy.

PTSD (post-traumatic stress disorder)—The recurrence of symptoms following a harrowing event, often including anxiety, nightmares, flashbacks, emotional detachment, and loneliness.

stem cell—An early precursor cell before it has developed all the hallmarks of the mature cell of a particular organ.

"Swamp Juice"—A nickname for the brown intravenous solution of the antifungal drug micafungin, sometimes protected from light during infusion by a brown bag.

"Van-Coke"—One nickname for hiding the very unpleasant flavor of the liquid form of the antibiotic vancomycin by chasing it with Coca-Cola.

Acknowledgments

Grateful acknowledgment is made to the editors of the following publications where these poems, some in altered form, first appeared:

American Journal of Nursing: "Poem for George"

Blood and Thunder: Musings on the Art of Medicine: "Awaiting Reconstitution," "Chemotherapy," "Please Define *Longer*"

Bloodletters Literary Magazine: "Rose Quartz Geode I Found in the Woods"

The Examined Life: A Literary Journal of the University of Iowa Carver College of Medicine: "Donor Search"

Families, Systems & Health: "MRI," "Waiting Room Waiting"

The Healing Muse: "Back Home, Day 459," "A Club for Those of Us Who Almost Died," "Victory Garden"

Inscape: "Cosmic Questions"

The Main Street Rag: "Feature Film: *Drug Study KEP DR78*," "For the Patients with Hair Loss," "PTSD"

New Limestone Review: "A Bag of Blood," "Demolition"

Pulse: "The Night Phlebotomist," "Seated on My Hospital Bed"

Reflective MedEd: "Doctor as Patient," "Maintenance Fatigue"

Snapdragon: A Journal of Art & Healing: "New Life"

The Somerville Times: "Choosing the Right Pumpkin, Farm Stand, Natick, Mass."

The Sunlight Press: "Retail Therapy"

Touch: The Journal of Healing: "An End to the Ends," "The
    Nurses There," "Skullcap," "Wanted: Lust"
The Worcester Review: "Drug-Induced Tendon Tear"

"The Hospital Mail" is published with permission of
JAMA, in which it first appeared.

"Bone Marrow Biopsy" and "With Feathers" are
published with permission of *JAMA Oncology*, in which
they first appeared.

"*Citrus aurantium*" was selected to appear as an example
of a response to a writing prompt in *The Practicing Poet:
Writing Beyond the Basics*, edited by Diane Lockward.
West Caldwell, NJ: Terrapin Books, 2018.

The book epigraph is from the poem "Before We Leave"
in *Lines of Defense: Poems* by Stephen Dunn. New York,
W. W. Norton & Company, Inc., 2014. Copyright © 2014
by Stephen Dunn. Reprinted by permission of W. W.
Norton & Company, Inc.

I want to express my enormous gratitude to Joan Cusack
Handler, publisher and founding editor of CavanKerry
Press, for her belief in this book. I am indebted as well
to her very special team for their editorial assistance
and production guidance. From the beginning, I have
relied on managing editor Gabriel Cleveland for his
calm reassurance and amazing proficiency with myriad
matters. Thank you, Joy Arbor, for your editorial
precision and gentleness; Dimitri Reyes, for your
patience translating the technical details of marketing;
and Ryan Scheife, for your thrilling gift of design. My
sincere thanks also to Baron Wormser for his honesty
and encouragement in the book's early days.

I am grateful to all those who helped me become a better poet along the way. Thank you, Joan Houlihan, for creating a climate to nourish my confidence as a poet. Jeffrey Levine, you stretched my vision for the poetry I could write and the book this could be. Although my workshops with Barbara Helfgott Hyett felt brutal early on, through the years she won my deep affection, adored my every return, and coaxed me to heartbreaking honesty. Thank you, Eric Hyett, for taking up my manuscript at "the table" to help my truth shine. How I appreciate my entire writing community in PoemWorks for their ever-present camaraderie and provocative suggestions! Special thanks, too, to Tom Daley for his skillful and perceptive tutelage, his exemplary readings, and his generous friendship and support of my work.

My life is enriched by my four offspring, who are always eager to receive a poem and ever enthusiastic about my pieces. I thank my sister for her sacrificial care during my convalescence, as well as her admiration, respect, and unqualified license to appear in my writing. Finally, I could not have captured this dream without the tireless advocacy of my beloved husband of more than four decades, my first and best reader, Ron.

Of course, I must acknowledge that I owe more than thank-yous to my principal oncologist, Dr. David Avigan, who has directed my lifesaving care amid a host of dedicated physicians, nurses, technicians, and therapists. Lastly, I give my immense gratitude to the young man whose stem cells allowed me the opportunity to live with the rich experiences and joys of my past nine years. Thank you for stepping forward at that Be The Match drive. As you have learned, Paul, our family loves you and celebrates you as our personal "Rock Star."

CavanKerry's Mission

A not-for-profit literary press serving art and community, CavanKerry is committed to expanding the reach of poetry and other fine literature to a general readership by publishing works that explore the emotional and psychological landscapes of everyday life, and to bringing that art to the underserved where they live, work, and receive services.

Other Books in the LaurelBooks Series

This book was printed on paper from responsible sources.

But I Still Have My Fingerprints was set in Karmina Sans,
a versatile and vivid sans serif font designed for setting
everything from short texts to long works requiring
extended reading. It was developed by Veronika Burian
and José Scaglione in early 2009.